Ruptured Quadder
Copyright © 2016 by Steven Gartner.

First Edition: March 2016

Contents

This book is dedicated to my parents. For their continued love, support and their ability to put up with my countless injuries I have incurred throughout my life.

Introduction

"You possibly have a Quadriceps Tendon Rupture." This was the initial assessment my Orthopedic Surgeon gave me when I was in his office back in 2007 when I suffered my first instance of what would become a very intimate injury and journey for me. "It's the same injury Bill Clinton recently had" my doc stated. I still had no idea what it was, but I knew it was serious.

Later that day I went online to look up former President Clinton's injury and became intrigued and wanted to learn as much about this injury as I could. However, I needed to be sure that this was the exact injury as my doctor stated and the only way to be sure was to have an MRI done on my right leg.

In the summer of 2007 I lost control of the Jet Ski that I was on and completely ruptured my right quadriceps tendon from my knee. It was the most painful injury that I have ever suffered in my life and believe me; I have been through a lot of injuries in my life time.

I quickly realized this was one of the most serious and longest healing leg injuries there is. When I was 6 years old I broke my femur while skiing in Austria and have always thought that was one of the worst injuries I had ever gone through. Boy how wrong I was.

Having gone through a rehabilitation process of what took around 18 months to fully be back to what I considered my normal self, I vowed to myself that I would never want to go through something like that again. Well wouldn't you know it, on January 6, 2013 while skiing at Stevens Pass east of Seattle, Washington I did the unthinkable.

I not only fully ruptured one of my quadriceps again, but I ruptured both of them resulting in an even worse injury than I experienced 6 years before.

I had incurred the dreaded Bilateral Quadriceps Tendon Rupture. With my previous research about this injury and my experience with my 2007 injury, I knew what was in store for me and what lied ahead in terms of recovery and rehab. I was devastated to say the least. I broke down and cried, but it was more of being in disbelief that how could I have possibly done this to myself again.

The following is my story of both of my accounts of injuring my quadriceps tendons and how I dealt with each injury and the process of rehabilitating my leg(s) and getting back to a normal life again. Initially I wanted to document my story much like others have, but once I got healed and recovered, I quickly put sharing my story on the backburner.

Fast forward six years and having to go through this injury again but this time with both legs, I really felt a strong desire to share both my stories because I knew people would benefit from my story. So I started a blog online to document both of my injuries and my story and share with other people who have gone or are currently going through this injury.

I know I benefitted from reading stories of people who have gone before me. Just reading another person's story and journey of getting back to normal was helpful and inspiring to me.

I hope you will find some real benefit from this book and I hope that I could share some useful advices that perhaps made life a little easier while going through this injury. If nothing else perhaps I can make dealing with your quad tear(s) a little more positive by sharing my stories with you and showing you that there is a light at the end of the tunnel.

With that I ask that you will reach out to me and share your story. And perhaps one day you will share mine and your story to another you may cross paths with that have also experienced the dreaded Quadriceps Tendon Rupture.

2007 Accident

It was a beautiful Saturday summer day in June of 2007 in my home town of Seattle. My buddy Mike had called me up early that morning and invited me to go boating. "Hell yea!" I said since you don't want to pass up a beautiful sunny day here in Seattle.

Looking back now, I wish I would have had something else planned that day or an excuse not to have made it. But... I met Mike at the usual spot for boating. He launched his boat at Coulon Beach located in Renton about 17 minutes southeast from Seattle.

It was early afternoon when we finally got the boat in the water, cracked open a beer and toasted to what should have been a gorgeous day ahead on the lake. Also joining us on the boat was my buddy photographer extraordinaire Darren.

As the day progressed Mike drove the boat to a popular area on Lake Washington called Juanita Beach located near Kirkland Washington. An hour or so passed when a friend of Mikes came into view in the distance on a jet ski. He got closer and tied up to us and came on board and mentioned the jet ski was free to use for anyone. I was eager to get on it and rip it up, but Darren beat me to it.

Darren was putzing around the lake trying to check out the local bikini girls dancing in the wake boarding boats when he finally made his way back to Mike's boat.

At this point I was so ready to get on the ski and cruise the lake. I took the life-vest from Darren and got on the jet ski and started to throttle up. It quickly became apparent to me that this was no ordinary jet ski or any one I have been on before. This one had power and lots of it.

I kept increasing the speed and soon I felt the true power of this wave-runner. It felt like I was doing 60 mph or more when I started feeling some loss of control. The water, which looked like glass on the surface, soon dissipated and big chop started setting in. I tried to absorb the shock of the chop by partially standing up on the jet ski, but I also continued to gain speed very quickly.

Why I didn't simply release the throttle still perplexes me to this day. I thought if I stood up part way I could absorb the shock with my bent legs/knees and keep my current speed and pace. Oh I wrong I was...

All I remember just before the accident was 1) I was traveling at an incredibly high rate of speed 2) I was starting to lose control and 3) how was I going to regain control of this jet-ski while traveling so fast and losing control.

Looking back now I realize that all I really had to do was to sit down, take my hand and off the throttle lever and let the ski slow down by itself. But it all happened so fast. The next thing I remember was that I tried to steer to the left in hopes of slowing the jet-ski down, and then I just remember being tossed in the air and into the water.

When I surfaced I remembered quite clearly a very severe and sharp pain in my right leg. When I was upright and somewhat buoyant in the water, I brought my right leg out of the water with great pain and noticed a big lump about 6 inches above where my knee cap should have been. I thought my knee had been shoved up towards my thigh. It was an excruciating pain just moving my leg a few inches.

All I remembered at that point was that my summer was done for and I had one very serious injury that would take a LONG time to heal. Oh that and I had no health insurance coverage at the time. So going broke also raced through my mind.

So there I was floating in Lake Washington with a very messed up leg and without any boats near me. I tried to get back on the jet ski but soon realized that even moving my leg an inch led to the most intense pain I have ever experienced.

After having tried several times to get back on the ski I realized that I needed to figure out another way to get back to my buddies. Thankfully I had a life vest on because floating in the deeper part of the lake with a severely injured leg and nothing to assist with keeping me a float, would have been extremely difficult and painful.

Knowing that I couldn't get back on the jet ski, my only other options were to either yell for help or try swimming back. Since I was close to the middle of the lake swimming back would have taken me forever and I realized that swimming away from the jet ski would have made me even less visible and possibly a target for a high speed boat running me over.

So I decided to stay put and started yelling from the top of my lungs for help. The only problem was that there were no boats near me and the boats

I could see in the distance were blasting music, killing any chance for someone to hear me.

After yelling for help for what felt like an hour, one boat that had drifted closer to me did finally hear me. I raised my arms waving back and forth and I remember seeing a gentleman on the boat nodding his head and he proceeded with starting up his boat.

When the boat finally got closer to me I noticed an elderly couple on board and the man called out to me asking me if I was OK. "I hurt my leg really bad and need to get to the hospital!" I shouted.

As the boat got closer to me the man shut off the motor and raced to the stern of the boat to help me up the ladder. That had to have been the most challenging steps I ever had to get up on since my right leg felt like a noodle and anytime it was bent even a fraction of a degree I felt the searing pain.

I managed to finally get into the boat to catch my breath and thank the couple for coming to my aid. I had advised them on what had happened to me.

The kind man started up the boat and proceeded to call 911 and off we went. I asked him if we could make a quick stop to where my friends were at, so I can tell them what had happened. When we came closer to where my friends were at I quickly told them what had happened, where the jet ski was and that I needed to get to the hospital ASAP!

Me and my new found rescuers were off to the main pier in Kirkland. During the boat ride the guy's wife, who happened to be a nurse, had some strong Motrin on hand and gave me a few. She also asked if I would like to 'numb' the pain with a swig of whiskey they had on board. Whiskey and powerful Motrin tablets? What a perfect combo to help kill my pain I thought.

So I took the Motrin and chugged them down with a healthy dose of Makers Mark. It took some time to get to the dock so I got to chat it up with my new boat mates for a bit. The man (damn I wish I could remember his name), told me that he was going to have open heart surgery soon. Hearing that made me just a bit more calmer inside knowing that although I just suffered a major leg injury, the situation could have always been much worse.

I would find out later that a newlywed couple died jet skiing a few weeks after my accident in the Seattle area which really hit home.

As we were nearing the dock I could already hear the ambulance siren nearby. Three Kirkland firefighter/paramedics arrived quickly at the scene and brought a stretcher. The biggest challenge was to lift me out of the boat.

Having a body weight of around 235+ pounds, lifting my big ass was enough of a challenge, but getting me out of that boat took extra special maneuvering since my leg had to be as straight as possible. Two of the firefighters secured my leg with a straight brace they had and then pulled the straps tight to ensure a secure fit.

After they carefully maneuvered me from the boat onto the stretcher they wheeled me to the ambulance. Being the photographer that he is, Darren took a few candid pictures that are posted on my blog. At that time, I was thinking why the hell is he taking photos of this event, but looking back now I'm glad he did. In a weird way it's nice to look back at these pics and recall the unfortunate event that had happened to me.

Once I was secured onto the stretcher I thanked the couple on the boat for helping me and providing me with booze and painkillers. I wished the elderly man best of luck with his upcoming open heart surgery. I wished I had gotten his contact info so we could have shared after stories. I hope he and his wife are doing well.

Inside the ambulance I was trying to make light of my accident with the paramedic who was inside with me by joking around. All I kept thinking about was what the hell did I do to my knee and so much for my summer.

I also had a date planned that evening so I had to call and tell her the situation. She felt terrible for me and I advised her that I'd be in touch later in the day and keep her posted on my situation. It was a quick ride from Kirkland to Overlake Hospital which is in the neighboring city of Bellevue less than 10 minutes away.

When I arrived at Overlake Hospital in Bellevue, Washington I was given some more pain medication and waited to get x-rays done to rule out any broken bones. After the x-rays were taken and assessed by the doctor, he confirmed to me that there was no broken bones.

He advised me to get an MRI since he felt it was a tendon rupture of some sort but he couldn't give me specifics. I was given a referral of a specialist and was sent on my way.

I quickly learned that I was unable to walk normally meaning I couldn't move my right leg forwards. I figured out that the only way that I could walk was and get around the ER was to walk backwards which was a sight all to its own. My parents had arrived soon after and the next challenge awaited me.

Since I had to keep my leg completely straight to avoid the pain, sitting in the front passenger seat was not an option. So I decided to lay down in the back of the car and advised my dad to lift my leg while I shimmied my way into the car keeping my leg as straight as possible as we proceeded to head back to where I parked my car.

When we got to my car my dad drove it back to my place while I kept my mom company since she was fearful of driving on the freeway at night. Once at my place I, with extreme difficulty, made my way up my stairs to my apartment. I said goodbye to my parents who would take me to the doctor's clinic a few days later for my MRI.

MRI & Surgery

I had to wait 3 days to get my MRI mainly due to availability. I figured it wasn't too long of a wait, however I had to wait 10 long days to get my surgery done which is far too long of a wait. The morning of the MRI my dad picked me up and drove me to the doctor's clinic in Bellevue and I had to wait a bit to get seen.

Once I hobbled into the room where the MRI machine was, I had to have the technician assist me with lifting my leg up but keep it completely straight. Any slight bend of the leg would result in excruciating pain. Once I got the leg in place and placed it into what looked like a clothes dryer, I had to keep it motionless in there for close to an hour.

Getting the results they said would take about a day and the doctor himself or the nurse would call with the details. But to my surprise I did get a call from the doctor and he stated what he initially thought was true, that I had fully ruptured my right quadriceps tendon. The doctor asked if I could come in the following day for more details as well as to schedule my surgery.

The next day I went back to the clinic and he again informed me the specifics of the injury, but he informed me that it was a fast procedure (under an hour) and I will be walking again normally in a few months.

I wasn't really sure how to take that news. I was glad the surgery would be quick and I wouldn't have to stay overnight or several days, but months to get back to normal walking concerned me. Not to mention having your leg in a brace completely straight for 6 weeks and then another 2 months or so in the brace to get my ROM (range of motion) back.

I arrived early to the hospital with my parents. My surgery was scheduled to be at 8 or so but I was advised that my doctor had another surgery before me and that he was running late. So my surgery was pushed forward around 2 hours.

After I got changed into the sexy hospital gown, the nurse came and got me all setup before I was going to talk with the anesthesiologist. My mom was in the room with me and we chatted for a bit and she had mentioned that they will most likely offer you a nerve block. She didn't steer me away from it but she did mention that there could be side effects from it. She had experienced side effects from one of her countless past surgeries.

The anesthesiologist came in. He was a young man probably around my age and he discussed what he would do while I had my surgery. He advised me of the nerve block and the decision rested in my hands, but he did mention that there are always chances of side effects but generally they were very minor.

For whatever stupid reason, I decided to decline the nerve block and boy, would I find out the hard way what a dumb decision that was. After I signed some forms to opt out of the nerve block I was quickly wheeled to the operating room where the fun was about to commence.

I remember very vividly how cold and sterile it felt in the room as they wheeled me. Blankets were placed on my upper body to keep me warm and then one of the nurses disinfected my skin with the ever popular orange dye called Povidone iodine.

Soon after my orthopedic surgeon showed himself and described what was going to happen during surgery. He placed his hand where the incision was going to happen and that he will anchor the tendon to the knee cap with sutures. "Done under an hour" he said. Then the anesthesiologist spoke briefly to me and asked me to count down from 100 and I remember reaching 96 or so and I was out like a light.

When I awoke I was so very groggy and all I remember was the nurse trying to help me from the stretcher onto the bed in the recovery room. All I remember doing was yelling loudly in excruciating pain. I swear to you it hurts to this day to think of it.

My mom was there advising the nurse to start giving me some pain medications and she, did but nothing seemed to help until I finally received some muscle relaxers which seemed to do the trick. That or all the meds combined finally kicked in and I was resting and I believe I was out for a bit.

I stayed in the recovery room for a few hours before it was time for me to be discharged. The next challenge was to get back into the back of my parents car which was a painful ordeal once before, but I managed since my dad kind of knew the protocol by lifting my leg up and keeping it completely straight. And then off we were to my parents' house in Monroe, Washington where I would spend the next 3-4 days to recover a bit from my surgery.

Femoral Nerve Block

I remember when I was all prepped for my first surgery back in 2007 and the anesthesiologist came into the room and discussed with me his role and on the procedure that was going to take place. After talking for a few minutes, the topic of whether I wanted to have a nerve block or not was the final question from him. I had remembered something my mother had mentioned about the possibility of having bad side effects from a nerve block.

The anesthesiologist mentioned that side effects could happen but is very rare now days. "Femoral nerve blocks are so commonly used in surgery this day and age, that very little goes wrong, but there is always that slight chance" he mentioned. Not wanting to take the risk of that 'slight chance', I made the decision to decline the nerve block, and all I can say now is, what an extremely bad decision that was!!!

Upon awakening after surgery all I can remember was how excruciating the pain was in my right leg. It felt like someone was stabbing me repeatedly in the leg with a knife. I was very groggy from the anesthesia and the more it wore off, the more pain I was experiencing. In all of my life, I have never experienced such intense pain as I did that morning in the recovery room.

My mom was telling the nurse to give me something to ease the pain but nothing seemed to work. The nurse gave me several different, highly-potent pain killers but there was no change in the pain level. Until sometime later, after having been giving some muscle relaxers, I was finally able to catch my breath. Even the initial injury itself wasn't this painful, probably since it was masked by adrenaline, fear and shock.

Fast forward five years, when I was in the same situation with having the same chat with the anesthesiologist, I made very damn sure to insist to him that I wanted the nerve block. However since both legs were damaged goods this time around, I was only able to get the nerve block on one leg. At first I was like "oh here we go again" and I made the decision (a good one this time) to get the block done on my left leg which was a complete-fully ruptured quad.

The nerve block lasted all day and night and kept my left leg numb until the following evening. The numbness wore off very gradually and while that was happening I was sure to be on my cocktail of painkillers and muscle relaxers.

So my advice to you on the day of the surgery after you have changed, been advised by the nurse, IV is in place, the time will come where the anesthesiologist will sit down and will ask you if you would like to have a nerve block to control the pain after you wake from surgery. Your answer should be "damn fricken straight I want a nerve block!!!" DO IT!!! I cannot stress this enough.

The pain after the first surgery to fix my right quad tendon in 2007 felt ten times worse than when I injured it on the lake jet skiing. When you think about the surgical procedure they have to perform to repair your leg(s) it makes sense of why it's so painful afterwards. The surgeon has to cut open your leg at the kneecap and pull the quad tendon and re-attach it to the knee cap. Doesn't sound so appealing does it?

When I was getting prepped for my surgery this past January, and I was talking with the anesthesiologist I made it a point to let him know that I wanted the nerve block. However, this time around I had two legs to deal with in terms of surgery and pain. Do I get it in the right leg or the left? I opted for the left since it was a full tear and I figured if the right leg has been through it before it couldn't be tougher the second time around LOL. What is so interesting is how very different the pain was this time around with my bilateral quadriceps tendon ruptures.

When I woke up I don't recall feeling any pain at all. I mean I knew the left leg was supposed to be fine and it was. Numb from my hip all the way down to my calf if I remember correctly. The nerve block as described to me was supposed to last between 10-14 hours, but actually it seemed to last much longer than that. I had surgery early morning and my left leg was numb and pain free until the following morning.

Now just because you are given a nerve block doesn't mean you will be pain free. Once the nerve block subsides the pain will slowly start to set in. However, the pain is managed with the healthy cocktail of pain med's that you will be prescribed from your doc and you will be taking the medication before the nerve block wears off.

After the Surgery

The next couple of days were very challenging since I had a cocktail of medications to take to keep the pain down and I had to remain stationary for the most part which is very hard for me to do. I remember how sleepy I would get with taking OxyContin and combined with the muscle relaxer I would be sleeping for hours a few times a day.

One of the things that happened to me frequently when I was fast asleep is that my injured leg would just jolt violently out of the blue and it would wake me right away and it was so very painful. I started to get worried that I might tear my sutures by doing this, but the doc advised me that this was normal and that as long as I wore my brace while sleeping, all would be good. Regardless of what the doc said, it still freaked me out every time it happened.

Many new challenges were ahead for me with this newly acquired injury and bathroom duties were definitely high on the list. Now I am not talking about peeing, that was fairly easy. I didn't think of using a pee bottle this time around so I always got out of bed to urinate and having the full brace made it easier than before. Before I always had to turn on my stomach and get out of bed that way since it was easier and safer as I didn't want to take a chance on bending the leg at all.

Going number 2 became quite challenging at first but I soon learned that as long as the injured leg stays straight, the other steps just required a little more movement so to speak LOL.

Another big challenge was being able to sleep normally while having this big brace around my leg. I quickly figured out and remember by reading other quadders stories that by placing a pillow or two in between your legs helps a ton that is if you are a side sleeper like me. When lying down flat on my back I would place a pillow under my knee and a few under my foot to elevate it a bit. I mainly did this when watching television or doing computer work.

My parents had two sets of stairs in their house but it didn't pose as much of a problem as it did for my 2013 bilateral injury. Having one good leg to put most of my weight bearing on made it very stable and easy to go down the stairs. Going down stairs is always a problem for quadders, not with going up at least that's been my experience. It's the whole bending of the knee thought that makes you cringe when navigating down the stairs when you have this injury since the last thing you want to do is re-injure the leg.

After my stint at my parents I had to get back home since I still had an online business to run. I had shipping labels to print and orders to pack and get to the post office. My dad helped out for the first few days but I got the hang of my new routine rather quickly. I was just a bit slower and a whole lot more cautious with moving around.

Life Adjustments

One of the first things I quickly realized after surgery was the adjustments one has to make with their daily routines. Getting in and out of bed, going to the bathroom, dressing oneself and bathing were tasks not normally thought about until this injury. The hardest part for me before the first surgery was getting out of bed. It was painful to try to get out of bed the normal way so I quickly learned that if I lie on my stomach and bring my leg out gravity would keep it straight which wouldn't have been the case the normal way.

Bathroom duties only became an issue with performing a number two. Now with a single quad rupture this was relatively still pretty easy and normal, but when you have a bilateral rupture it takes a bit of shifting ones upper body to make the process go smoothly.

I wasn't allowed to take a shower for the first few weeks since the doctor strongly advised against the sutures getting wet. So what I did instead was to take baths – "Calgon take me away" lol. I would prop one leg up and in the case for my bilateral tears, I propped both legs up so the sutures would be above the water line. I had to first get in the tub which by far was the most difficult part. Once in, I turned the water on and then propped up both my legs.

Getting dressed was pretty straight forward. I just had to make sure my legs were as straight as possible when putting on pants. The easiest way I found to do this is simply lay the pants on the floor with both leg openings spread wind enough for me to just place each foot in each opening. Then I would reach down and pull up my pants.

Of course some flexibility is required here so it would work just as well lying on the bed or floor and after you pull your pants over your legs you simply apply your leg brace(s).

One point I wanted to address that I mention in my blog and I also created a YouTube video about, was how you maneuver up and down a staircase. If you have stairs to deal with like I did on both occasions they can be very challenging especially going down them. Dealing with just one rupture, stairs were challenging but not impossible. Dealing with two quad ruptures proved to be a very daunting task. I had to figure out a way to navigate going down my stairs without fear or a possible accident.

I remember when I first ruptured my tendon and I was coming out of the ER and I was unable to walk forwards because of the pain and non-functioning quad. So I just decided to start walking backwards and it worked. So this came to me when I was looking down my stairs one day. I said "why don't I try walking down them backwards".

And it was a miracle how easy it was to walk backwards down my staircase. It was so much easier than getting on my butt and carefully sliding down them.

This was the case with many other little daily tasks that required a little tweak here and there to make life easier while I was rehabilitating my legs.

Physical Therapy

I believe it was at the 8 or 9 week mark that I was given the thumbs up to begin my PT. The doctor gave me a list of several qualified and recommended therapists in my area and I chose one at random I believe. It turned out that my random choice (this time) was a great choice.

My PT was a petite gal from Canada who was amazing. She wasted no time in putting me through some tough sessions that would get me back to normal movement as quickly as possible. I stayed with her for a few months before I went out on my own doing rehabilitation and strength conditioning at my local gym.

Some of the exercises that I felt helped tremendously were the bosu ball, wobble board, machine hack squat and light leg extensions. Aggressive leg stretches also really help although they were extremely painful in the beginning.

The road to recovery from leaving my Physical Therapist to where I was somewhat of a normal and abled-bodied person took some time. The hardest challenge was getting my leg to have a ROM of 90 degrees and then past 120. Once you get past that it will just be a matter of time with strengthening and continuing your stretching (very important) that you will be back to your normal self.

Being that I didn't have to be at a typical 9-5 job for this injury I could focus on my recovery a whole lot more than my later incurred injury. My daily routine consisted of going to the gym to do strength training, cardio, and I would utilize the pool to do my walking.

At home I would focus on stretching and isometric exercises. I eventually dropped the pool walking sessions when I could fully utilize the stationary bike as well as the treadmill.

Weight training consisted of very light one-legged leg extensions, machine leg presses, leg curls, abductor and adductor leg machines. I didn't consider doing any kind of squat movement until much later say at 7 or 8 months post-surgery. I realize light squats would have been ok to do, but something about the movement just made me feel very uneasy and I wasn't looking to get the muscle size I once had back. I just wanted to get my range of motion as close to normal as before and strength back so I could partake in my favorite physical activities like snow skiing, roller blading, scuba diving and hiking.

I really feel that this consistent daily training plan led to a faster recovery then if I wasn't exercising as frequent. I should point out that I did take the weekends off from weight training. I believe variety in movement is important so I didn't want to be stuck with always doing the same thing.

So on weekends I would try to walk around a local lake or some other popular spots around the Seattle area (weather dependent of course). The last thing I wanted to do is slip on wet pavement and re-injure myself.

ROM

ROM or Range of Motion is a very common topic brought up by quadders and rightfully so. Getting back one's range of motion is on the top of the list when you succumb to a quadriceps tendon rupture. When you literally go from a full ROM of perhaps 140 degrees or more (as pictured) to having a ROM of just a few degrees after surgery, you better believe it is on the high priority list for us.

From the onset of your injury, you quickly realize that any degree of bending the leg results in a very intense pain that makes you quickly want to straighten your leg to avoid the agony.

When you have your 2 week follow up with your Orthopedic Surgeon and you are advised and prescribed your new leg brace, your OS will go over the next 6-8 week plan of ROM with you using this new brace.

Now every OS will probably offer different suggestions via the use of the brace, but the plan for me on both occasions for my injuries was to increase my ROM range via my leg brace by 20%

every 2 weeks. My doc set the initial setting at 20 degrees so by the end of 6 weeks I was supposed to be at around 80 degrees of ROM although I was always a little more than that. I would say I was close or right at 90 degrees at the six week point.

At my follow up I was given the green light to start physical therapy the following week which of course excited the hell out of me. As before, I saw it as another little victory in my timeline of progress and of getting back to normal.

I would like to stress that everyone who is or has suffered a QTR will experience different rates of recovery speeds. You can't force your body to recover faster than it will allow itself to and nor should you. Don't make the mistake of being in a rush to get better. You will be back to normal or perhaps as close to normal soon enough, but it is going to take some time - quite a bit of time to be honest. So be smart and safe about your rehab and recovery phase of this injury.

The first 6 weeks is always the toughest with QTR. The 20 to 80 degree ROM is the hardest to reach and will seem to take forever, but once you reach 90 degrees and beyond the recovery time is much faster. You might have some sticking points for a while at certain ranges like I did. I think the hardest for me is to get past the point where you can fully move the pedals on a stationary bike. In the beginning every time I would try to ride one, I would just move the pedals back and forth as far as I could. The hardest part was to do a full rotation when I was just below the 90 -110 degree range. However once I got past that point my ROM increased very quickly.

I feel the stationary bike, whether standard as pictured above or a recumbent style is a perfect exercise to work on your ROM for your injured QTR(s). As I have mentioned elsewhere within this website, exercises such as swimming and walking in a pool are fabulous exercises for helping you get back your initial ROM, but the stationary bike should not be overlooked and is a fantastic piece of cardio equipment to re-gain a really broad ROM for your leg.

Driving Difficulties

T here were a few things the doctor didn't advise me on when I was in his office getting assessed about my injury. He probably suspected that I would figure them out as time went on or that I would ask him at a later date. One of the main concerns I had was when can I start driving again.

When I incurred my injury in 2007 I had landed a job a few days prior to the accident. I was supposed to start a few days after my surgery. Having been advised by my doctor soon after surgery that I wasn't supposed to drive for several weeks, I became very stressed out on what to do about my situation.

I brainstormed on how I could get to work. The job was computer support so I would be sitting all day which was something I could do, but how was I going to get to the job. My parents lived in Monroe and my friends all worked jobs so taxiing me around was not an option. It turned out that I didn't let my employer know soon enough about surgery and such and so I was basically let go from a job I didn't even start. Oh well, probably for the better I said. I still had my eBay business to bring in daily income so all was good in my book. My recovery was my primary importance. However, the extra income from this job would have helped with the medical expenses I incurred since I didn't have any medical insurance.

So what I did was to focus on my internet business and the rehabilitation of my leg. The one main hurdle I had to deal with was that with my internet business where I needed to go to the post office to drop off my orders and I had to do this several times a week if not daily. I knew about USPS pickup service request, but unfortunately that didn't apply to international orders and 70% of my business was international.

In the beginning my father helped out with taking me to the post office to drop off my orders, but I couldn't ask him to continue to do that since he was coming all the way from Monroe. I didn't really have friends that were readily accessible so I decided to go against the docs orders and figure out a way to drive myself.

Driving itself wasn't such a big issue, getting into my SUV was. My ride was, and still is a 2001

Nissan Xterra. It has been a wonderful car for me and this year I will have had it for over 10 years. Now the Xterra sits high off the ground so getting my right leg in was a bitch especially since it had to remain as straight as possible.

In the beginning I would try to lift the leg up and into the car but there were a lot of painful moments. I finally figured out that using a small towel or bandanna to wrap and lift up my brace and get my leg in was the ticket. Then I realized that I needed my butt to be lifted a little bit higher so my leg could remain straight without it being an issue to drive and also so it wouldn't be painful.

So I figured a pillow or something under my butt to sit on would elevate me and help make my leg straighten out and as I suspected, it worked out perfectly. I sat higher which straightened out my leg and I was now able to drive. Now bear in mind that this worked for me because my car had an automatic transmission. If you have a manual transmission it is going to be quite another story I am sure there is a work-a-round since all you really need is your feet to shift and brake, but I can't be sure since my experience was with an automatic. As long as your leg is straight all should be OK is what I suspect.

Now please understand, I am not condoning driving while injured, however sometimes you need to do what needs to be done especially if you have no other choice or workarounds. If you are in the position of having someone to help and do your daily tasks, then you have it made. But for some of us, like me who didn't have easy access to help, you have to make do with other ways. And sometimes 'other' ways is the only way possible.

Looking back now driving while being in my leg brace really wasn't that big of a deal. It was more of a morality issue because I felt I was going against doctors' orders, but I didn't do any harm to my leg(s) so all was ok.

Leg Braces

When the quadriceps tendon is fully ruptured you will experience a leg that is basically limp. You will not able to move your leg straight up when the tendon is completely torn. There is no anchor for the tendon so you have limp noodle so to speak. As mentioned many times before, quad ruptures come in many varieties. Some people have been able to move and walk for a bit with the torn tendon, others like me were unable to move at all.

Until you have your tendon repaired via surgery, the only way you can make any kind of necessary movements is to have your leg(s) locked in place and that is with a high quality leg/knee brace. Usually you are given one from the ER if that is where you went right after your accident, or you received it at your first doctor's visit when you get assessed and scheduled for your MRI. Unfortunately the leg braces you first receive are not high quality. They are subpar even though they do work well enough to get you by; until surgery that is.

It is usually at your 2 week Post-op visit to your doctor that he will issue (sell) you a retractable ROM adjustable leg brace. These are of very high quality and often times very expensive if you buy them from the doctor's office.

As I mention in my blog, do not buy the brace(s) from your doctor's clinic. They will sometimes be five times or more than the price you can get them for online. I remember the first brace I bought had a price tag of around $250 or more. Had I looked online beforehand I could have found countless of styles at a price hovering around $35-$50 and usually with free shipping. With sites like eBay and Amazon you will be able to find a fantastic high quality brace that is brand new with a price that doesn't break the bank.

Obviously I didn't think about this in the beginning when I suffered my first quad rupture. Since I wasn't aware what was needed for rehab and recovery I just went with the flow. But fast forward to my second experience of my bilateral injury I knew for the most part on what was in store and what lied ahead for me.

Medical Costs

I went through my medical files a while back and I came across my old statement from my first surgery repair in 2007. It was interesting to see the differences in cost from my first quadriceps rupture to the bilateral rupture I incurred years later. As you can see from the image below, the first time I had a 'suture tendon' repair done the cost was $1,572. Now mind you, this was only the cost to repair my tendon. Additionally there were bills for the anesthesiologist, the hospital, and physical therapist.

Having had no insurance during my first injury was costly indeed. I was unemployed at the time and without any medical coverage so I started to stress on the bills that had come my way soon after my surgery. I was advised however, that being in the position I was in I could write a hardship letter to get my medical costs greatly reduced. To my surprise it worked very well.

If I remember correctly my anesthesiology bill was reduced from over $1,000 down to around

$600 and my hospital stay was reduced from $7,000 down to almost half that amount. Unfortunately my surgery cost and the MRI was not reduced. Oh well, you can't win them all right?

Fast forward to 2013 and my surgery costs are almost $4,000 dollars more since I ruptured both quads, even though the right leg was only a partial tear. I'm just thankful I had some good insurance to cover most of the surgery fee. However, since my insurance deductible wasn't met, I was responsible for around $1,500 for the difference. The anesthesia charge was $1,200 and was reduced to $192 with insurance adjustments.

The hospital stay was close to the same cost as my previous stay in 2007 which I found odd. I'm still in shock on how a short stay of less than half the day can run over seven grand. Thankfully the bulk of that fee was covered again by my insurance.

2013 Accident

I remember when I suffered my first quad tendon rupture and reading Jim's account of his bilateral injuries and I said to myself "I cannot imagine having both of my quad's torn!" Dealing with one full tear was an awful experience for sure, but dealing with two of them? Unreal I thought. With one tear at least you still have a good leg to bear weight on while babying the injured leg. I never suspected my worst nightmare would one day become a reality.

The date was January 6th 2013, a date I will always remember as having suffered the worst possible injury. I was skiing with my friend Jill at Stevens Pass a very popular ski destination in Washington State. It was a Sunday morning and conditions were just about perfect for carving some turns. I had been waiting for a few weeks to ski my first day of the season due to crappy conditions the past month.

I had brought my Go Pro that day to get some footage of us skiing but decided to leave it in the car when we arrived and my plan was to get it later in the day. I wanted to get some good runs in beforehand. Looking back now, although it would have been tough to watch in one respect, I could have had actual footage of my accident and what had happened before and after the fact.

Jill and I were only on the mountain for a mere 2 runs before I suffered my accident. We decided to do a warm up run on Skyline which is a good intermediate to advanced run that covers a good area of the mountain. After that we figured why not take it up a notch and take skyline up again and shoot over to 7th Heaven to take advantage of the new fresh deep powder. So we did and the run was amazing.

So just to back track a bit, I have been skiing since I was 4. So I consider myself a pretty good skier. Stevens Pass' 7th Heaven is considered a very advanced route or a double diamond. We both navigated this route without problems and it wasn't until I decided to take my old 'high school' route of skiing under the old blue jay chair and then go ski near Daisy and back to Skyline to do it all over again.

It was incredible skiing up to that point coming down the mountain. Skiing under where the old blue jay chair used to be, I decided to ski over to the Daisy lift (a bunny run) and decided to get a bit of air time from the jumps that are to the right of the chairlift. I decided to avoid the first jump since it can really launch a person and if you didn't know what the landing was like beforehand, it could be a terrible end result. So I skipped that jump and skied down a few moguls and took the next jump.

The jump I took wasn't really that big looking as I was skiing towards it. It probably got me off the ground 6 or 7 feet, but it was the landing that sealed my fate. What looked soft and full of fresh powder from the distance was a landing that was completely flat and hard. Having less than optimum ski goggles and skiing in the bright daylight also gave me a false sense of perspective. Add to that, my ski bindings were set to the highest setting preventing you to easily pop out of them which can be very helpful if you ski a lot of deep powder.

Of course the flip side is that since you don't pop out of your bindings easy, you risk a higher chance of injuries to the legs. This was the result with my incident.

What I remember was that I went off the jump and as soon as I landed I felt and heard a loud thud.

I face planted hard and my left ski came off. Everything from that point seemed to move in slow motion. I felt dizzy and I knew something was wrong. I still had my right ski on and felt a sharp pain in my right knee. I turned around and noticed I was sitting somewhat on my right ski. I tried to straighten out my leg but couldn't so I used my hands to release the ski from my binding.

I soon gained some clarity for a bit and knew I was badly hurt but I couldn't tell right away what was injured. I tried to stand up but realized I couldn't and that's when I started freaking out.

Being right under the Daisy chairlift people above me would call out and ask me if I was alright. Jill shouted back that I wasn't and if they could notify the ski patrol for help. I was just sitting there confused with what felt like shock setting in.

It wasn't long at all until the first ski patroller came to the scene. He had walked towards us and said that he saw me 'bite it'. As he came closer to me he asked where I was hurt. I started feeling dizzy again and my body started shaking, telling me and the ski patroller that I was slowly going into shock.

Trying to keep my composure and some sense of humor I told him in detail what had just

Steven Gartner

happened to me. He asked me where I was hurting and what my pain level was. At that point I didn't really feel much pain at all probably due to the shock setting in. I advised him that I couldn't stand up or lift my legs.

The ski patroller radioed for backup and soon after another ski patroller was on the scene. They had me lay down straight and relax as they secured me in the red blanket you see in the pics and a few minutes after that the third ski patroller showed up with the infamous toboggan.

Now just like my accident in 2007, I find it ironic that yet again I had three rescue personnel assist in securing me and placing me in the stretcher/toboggan. Apparently my big ass is heavier than normal and needs three adult males to lift and move it LOL.

As I was getting tobogganed down the mountain thoughts of anger, frustration, and regret filled my mind. "How can I have been so stupid," I kept thinking and "why do I get injured so often." Looking back now I realize though the situation could have been much worse. I could have broken my neck or injured my spine and have been paralyzed.

The site of the accident could have also been worse. I could have injured myself at the top of 7th Heaven which would have made it very hard for the ski patrollers to secure and get me into the toboggan and down the double diamond run. I quickly realized self-pity, anger, resentment and such all though have their normal place in a situation such as this, but it just doesn't make it any better.

When I reached the ski patrol hut there were already quite a few people in there with injuries. Two ladies had twisted their knees and another one was just a little banged up. To my surprise, there were two doctors there who volunteered their time and expertise. One was an orthopedic surgeon who, after I was done talking with the head ski patrol, assessed my injuries and immediately could tell what I had done to my left leg. He placed his finger just above my left knee cap and could feel the gap. "Yes just as I suspected. You have a full quad tendon rupture" he said.

When I heard those words I just froze and my mouth dropped. All I could think about at that moment was what I endured 5 years before and how long it took to heal my previous quad rupture.

I looked at Jill and I just shook my head and said "oh god no, not again!" I was so angry at myself as to how I could have possibly incurred this injury again, and possibly to both legs. The OS however, wasn't able to asses my right leg. I was able to lift my right leg when fully straightened out and there wasn't such a noticeable gap above my right knee cap. So he thought it was possibly a partial tear, but I would need to get an MRI done to get specifics of the injury. I was given pain medication and both of my legs where put in temporary braces.

Now I had to call my parents but I didn't want them to know right away what had happened. I wanted to just speak to my brother and have him meet me at my house. I didn't want my parents to worry especially since they were part of my first ordeal in 2007. I spoke with my bro and told him what had happened and to meet at my house.

Little did I know that my mom was listening in on the other line. She called me back and told me she was listening in and asked me what had happened. I just broke down at that point and felt so angry at myself since I knew my parents would be involved yet again after surgery.

After I signed all the paper work and was given the OK to leave the ski patrol hut, the once again difficult part of transporting me and lifting me took place. Jill was going to drive my SUV while I had to lie in the back seat. As I remembered from my prior quad tear, I had to lay down with my legs completely straight otherwise severe pain would be felt. It was quite the process to get me out of the wheelchair and into the back of my Xterra. Once resting somewhat comfortably in the back Jill started driving us back to my place.

Here We Go Again

The first time I broke down with resentment and frustration was at the ski hut where the volunteer orthopedic surgeon assessed my situation. The second time I broke down was when I arrived back home from Steven's Pass with my friend Jill where my brother was waiting and my parents would soon arrive.

My parents had made previous plans to take my brother out for dinner since he was flying back home to Oklahoma the very next day. Since I wasn't able to join them I stayed at my house. That's when it really hit me. I was just in such disbelief that I had done this again and it was twice as bad and I knew what lied ahead for me.

I guess looking back I felt worse for my parents because that look in their eyes when they met me and Jill at my house and I could just tell my dad was looking at me like "why are you till acting and doing crazy things a 20 year old would do".

When my brother arrived back from dinner he mentioned that he would delay his flight out by a couple of days so that he could assist me with my situation. I was beyond thrilled since it took my parents out of the equation and it took the burden off of them. I thanked my brother over and over again and we proceeded to have some drinks. And then we had some more which at the time helped heal numb the pain and disappointment I was feeling for the rest of the night.

My brother stayed with me for a few days. Just long enough to ferry me to and from the MRI, surgery, and post-surgery. He helped out with walking my dogs since that having them was something I didn't have to contend with back in 2007.

In terms of my dogs, I felt at the initial post-surgery recovery phase that it would be best to have my good friend of mine watch over them for a couple of weeks while I heal up and get more ROM in my legs. She ended watching them for over 3 weeks which was such a big help. I felt it was better for me and my dogs (who I absolutely love dearly). The last thing I would want is to trip over one of them while navigating the stairs or such.

Another MRI & Surgery

With a repeat injury I knew what was in store. Another lengthy MRI, however now it would be done on both quadriceps tendons. I was also looking at receiving another surgery to fix my tendons. There was still uncertainty on the severity of my right leg, but my left quad was definitely a full tear as diagnosed by the Volunteer Orthopedic Surgeon at the ski pass.

As luck would have it, I was able to get my MRI done two days later with the surgery following the very next morning. I was so relieved that I could get it all done back to back instead of waiting over a week as was the case with my first injury back in 2007. The MRI appointment was scheduled at 4pm and it would take around 45 minutes per leg. Thankfully this MRI machine allowed you to lay down completely unlike the previous one I had used where you just placed your leg into a giant tube like contraption.

Once my MRI was complete, my brother who had waited for me patiently, drove us back home and I rested and mentally prepped for the surgery the following day. As per instructions previously given to me by the nurse, I was supposed to fast for around 12 hours prior to my surgery. Fasting wasn't really hard to do since the pain medications I was taking killed my appetite. Luckily for me my mom had some strong pain killers on hand that I used and tied me over until I could get a prescription of some others after surgery.

Surgery was scheduled for the very next day at 7:30 am with a check in one hour prior. I remember with my first surgery of being on the hospital stretcher and getting wheeled into the operating room. It felt so very cold and sterile in there.

The same orthopedic surgeon who assessed and performed surgery on me back in 2007 did so also in 2013. I figured he was very experienced and he knew my history so who better to take care of me the second time around.

My doctor walked into the surgery room and advised me on what was about to take place via the bilateral quad tendon surgery. He advised me that it would take about one and a half hours to two hours, if memory serves me right. Then I remember the anesthesiologist telling me to count down from 100 while the anesthesia kicks in. I believe I made it to about 95 and I was out. This time around everything seemed similar except for the counting down part.

The other big difference this time around was when I woke up from surgery. This time it was no real issue at all meaning I had virtually no pain whatsoever. Unlike my previous post-surgery experience where I was screaming like a banshee, the nerve block did its thing for my left leg and I felt very little pain in my right leg. That by far was the biggest relief for me as I vividly remember how excruciating it was when I woke up after surgery back in 2007.

It took a few hours before I was given the approval to be discharged and let my brother drive me home. I was surprised however, that I didn't stay overnight like some quadders who have had a bilateral surgery done. I've read stories from people where some have stayed in the hospital for a few days to a week or more for post-op recovery. I assume every hospital has different rules and procedures. Now that I had the surgery done, the real fun was about to begin and by that I mean the rehab and recovery phase.

Tips & Tricks

Rupturing ones quadriceps tendon is a completely different experience. At least for me it was and I have been through the gambit of injuries. I suffered numerous sprained ankles, broken nose, broke my femur, rotator cuff and more. But none really compared to the lifestyle changing quad rupture because with this injury you had to adapt and find new ways to do normal everyday tasks.

Walking, toilet use, bathing, getting dressed and even getting out of bed take on a whole new meaning of becoming creative to accomplish these everyday routines. So by having gotten creative over the years with my two injuries I have devised this list of tips and tricks that were helpful for me and hopefully can be of some use to others.

Femoral Nerve Block

As I have mentioned before in this site, make sure you agree on getting the Nerve Block from the Anesthesiologist when he/she sits down with you before the surgery. I can't stress this enough. Unless you have some condition that prevents you from receiving this - GET IT!

Telescopic ROM Hinged Knee Brace(s)
Purchase your leg brace(s) online via Amazon or eBay to save quite a bit of money. If you buy your brace from the doctor's office expect to pay a hefty amount. If I remember correctly
insurance didn't cover the cost of the brace, but I could be wrong or this might have changed.

Experienced Physical Therapist
Don't just settle for one that was advised to you by your doctor. Make sure you seek out a qualified and experienced physical therapist that has experience with quad tendon ruptures. If he/she does not find another one. Don't waste your time and money on a PT that has no knowledge of this type of injury and if they do find out how many clients they have dealt with previously.

Also make sure they are putting you through exercises and rehabilitation procedures that will benefit your injury in the short term. What I mean here is make sure they are not dragging the rehab process out for an unnecessary period of time. I know some physical therapists who work like chiropractors and keep prolonging what will really help you and just try to get you to keep coming back and back and back.

Gym membership

If you don't already have a membership to a health club or gym get one. Preferably one with access to a pool and a hot tub. These will help with your rehabilitation profoundly as water therapy is amazing physical therapy for a ruptured quad tendon. The late night sessions of walking in the pool from one end to the other worked wonders for my legs and I believe also cut my recovery time down. The other benefits of a gym will be access to strength training equipment and cardio machines.

Walk down the stairs backwards

If you are unfortunate enough to live by yourself with this injury as I was and you live in a 2 story or more apartment or house, then navigating the stairs is extremely scary and tricky. Now if you have only one QTR it is still manageable to walk down the stairs with no problems, but when you have 2 full length leg braces... forget about it! Walking down the stairs backwards was the only method I could use to get down the stairs without sliding down.

Car Cushion

Driving was a necessity for me since I ran an online business and needed to get to the post office. Getting out of the house helped to clear the head and not feel like a hermit. For me a properly placed cushion or pillow lifted my driving position enough to wear I could keep my brace straight. This also applies if you are the passenger and need to keep the leg straight. Of course I should mention that your height will have a lot to do with this as long legs will make it more difficult for driving. If you are short you probably will be OK without the cushion.

MRI & Surgery

When I first ruptured my right quad tendon back in 2007 I knew absolutely nothing about this injury until my OS advised me that it was the same injury Bill Clinton suffered (although his was a partial tear). I quickly researched online about this injury and found out that the sooner you have surgery performed the better outcome will be for your injury. I had to wait over a full week for my first QTR injury, but my second occurrence I got scheduled in just a few days. Getting the surgery done as quickly as possible means you are on the road to recovery sooner.

Reaching/Grabbing tool

There were countless of times I could have used one of these, but I never got around to getting one. Get one ahead of time for it will come in handy when you least expect it.

Pee Bottle

This can really help out especially in the beginning soon after you had surgery. Getting out of my bed was very difficult especially since I had a very tall bed frame. Those mid night pee sessions and the pain in the ass to get out of bed just to pee with 2 leg braces can be quickly resolved with a pee bottle placed close by.

Stay Positive

Along with getting the Nerve Block, I can't stress being and staying positive enough. It is completely natural and expected to get depressed, angry, and resentful after your incur this injury. You will probably go hrough periods of 'why me?', 'if only I would have done this', etc. Save the pity party for another time. I don't want to sound like a dick, but being negative and down on yourself does nothing for your recovery. Instead, make and keep timeline recovery goals such as this week my ROM increased by this percentage amount' or 'next week I get my stitches out' etc.

Track your progress

Keep track of your progress whether in your head, a journal, or better yet post it online. I wish I had done a step by step and posted all my progress, thoughts, etc. as they happened like I originally wanted to because now I have to backtrack and recollect on certain parts of what happened and share it online.

Share your experience

It might sound odd, but I felt really good when I talked about and shared my experience with tearing my quad tendons. The more I talked about it the better I felt. I'm not sure why, but just sharing my story gave me a little confidence booster and even more so if saw another person at the gym going through the same thing. Try it, you might surprise yourself.

Disabled Parking

W hen you have your 2 week follow up with your OS, make sure you get your temporary disabled parking application form from him/her. Also make sure the form is signed, dated and if you can get the maximum 'privilege duration' marked off the better. In Washington State it is 6 months and a sample application is shown below:

This parking permit will help out a lot in the course of your injury especially in the beginning phase of your recovery. I'm not trying to advocate laziness by taking advantage of being able to park closer, but you will be spending enough time with rehab via physical therapy, gym, and/or some other form of strength and conditioning for your leg(s). I mean really! You just went or are going through one of the worst leg injuries that can be endured so a little convenience here and there is deserved. Besides, driving will be challenging enough.

The disabled parking permit was a huge help for me this time around since I have two dogs to take for their daily walks, and having found an off-leash dog park near my area that had disabled access was such a relief. Let me tell you, walking two dogs with two leg braces is very difficult and oh did I mention, not very safe? I didn't want to take a chance of re-injuring my legs yet again.

Also with my new job I started, taking the bus wasn't an option in the beginning since the bus stop was quite a long ways away from my office and there were a few areas that had quite the steep downhill walk. I didn't want to take a chance with walking downhill especially the first 6 weeks after surgery when your leg braces are locked straight. So parking in the employee handicap stall was a huge bonus.

By the time your parking permit expires your leg(s) should have rehabilitated enough that driving shouldn't be a problem anymore. Your ROM after the 6 month mark should be way past 90 degrees. Of course everyone's rate of recovery is different so there might be quadders who might not be at the range of motion that allows for driving.

QTR Terms

Here is a list of frequently used terms that you will hear associated with quadriceps tendon rupture:

- BQTR
  - Bilateral Quadriceps Tendon Rupture
- FWB
  - Full Weight Bearing
- MRI
  - Magnetic Resonance Imaging
- OS
  - Orthopedic Surgeon
- PT
  - Physical Therapy
- QUADDER
  - A person who has experienced a ruptured quadriceps tendon or bilateral rupture
- QTR
  - Quadriceps Tendon Rupture
- RQT
  - Ruptured Quadriceps Tendon
- ROM
  - Range of Motion

Reflecting Back

Looking back, now that it has been just over 3 years since my bilateral accident and 9 years since my first quad tear, I have to say that it's hard to fathom that I went through two instances of this serious injury. What's even harder to accept at times is how the hell I got to be so reckless to have this happen to me twice.

But like anything else, you cannot dwell on the past and feel sorry for one self. Things happen, some say for a reason and perhaps my reason was to endure this injury twice so I can share my story with others who are or will go through with this in the future.

I will say that I now take a whole heck of a lot more precaution when doing physical activities. I really have a better appreciation of what all I went through in terms of rehabilitation with physical therapy, walking and living life temporarily with locked leg braces and just doing everyday tasks.

One thing has remained however, and I'm not talking about those gorgeous scars. No, the one thing that remains is my eagerness to talk and share about my experience of this injury. When I meet others and/or chat with fellow quadders online, I get passionate about this topic with others because in the realm of injuries, QTR is still somewhat of a rare injury to receive.

Once you experience this injury you get a real intimate connection and appreciation of what all you went through. And the connection and appreciation becomes even stronger when you go through it a second time.

With that, I will say goodbye for now. I truly hope you enjoyed reading my story and I hope you got something out of it. Perhaps you are not just a curious reader, but a fellow quadder and so I encourage you to share your story with others as so many other quadders have.

If nothing else, shoot me a quick message and share your story with me. Reach out to me via my blog online at www.QuadTendonTear.com and I look forward to hearing from you.

To be continued...

Continue the story by following
'Scuba' Steven Gartner on his blog:

Quad Tendon Tear:
http://www.QuadTendonTear.com

Connect with me on Facebook:
https://www.facebook.com/ScubaDubaDoo

If you liked this book, please leave
me a positive review on
Amazon.

Made in the USA
Middletown, DE
03 September 2016